Endocrine system

Balance

3 Underrated Tips To Balance

Your Hormones

JENNIFER VARGAS

Table of Contents.

<u>*Chapter 4.*</u>

<u>*How Can I Help Keep My Endocrine System Healthy Naturally?*</u>

<u>*When Should I Call the Doctor?*</u>

<u>*why is the endocrine system slow?*</u>

The following procedures would be performed during a proper evaluation to find an endocrine issue in a child: 1) A physical examination to gauge the size and shape of endocrine glands; 2) A blood test to gauge hormone levels; 3) Imaging tests like an ultrasound or MRI to view the endocrine glands; and 4) Urine tests to gauge electrolyte levels. A full genetic testing panel may also be beneficial to explore genetic abnormalities that can cause endocrine difficulties. Finally, genetic counseling may help evaluate environmental and family history aspects that contribute to endocrine issues.

Chapter 1.

what is the endocrine balance.

The body's synthesis and secretion of hormones, which are chemical messengers that control numerous bodily processes like growth, metabolism, reproduction, and stress response, are regulated by the endocrine system, a complex network of glands and organs.

The appropriate operation and communication of the various elements of the endocrine system are referred to as the endocrine balance.

The production and release of hormones occur in the proper amounts and at the proper periods when the endocrine system is in balance. Maintaining good health and preventing diseases depend on this equilibrium. Genetics, lifestyle choices, drugs, and underlying medical issues are just a few of the causes of hormonal imbalances.

These imbalances can cause a variety of symptoms, such as fatigue, weight gain or loss, mood swings, and problems with reproduction.

A healthy lifestyle, including frequent exercise, a balanced diet, and enough sleep are necessary to maintain endocrine balance. Moreover, reducing stress and avoiding pollutants in the environment helps enhance endocrine function. See a healthcare provider for a diagnosis and treatment options if you think you may have an endocrine imbalance.

Balance endocrinology.

A balanced endocrine system, which is in charge of producing and secreting hormones, is referred to as having balanced endocrinology. Hormones are chemical messengers that control some body processes, including development, metabolism, reproduction, and stress response. The maintenance of overall health and the prevention of many illnesses depends on a balanced endocrine system.

Hormones are created and released in the proper amounts and at the proper times when the endocrine system is in equilibrium. However, abnormalities in hormone secretion and production can arise as a result of several variables, including underlying medical disorders, lifestyle choices, drugs, and heredities. Many symptoms, including exhaustion, weight gain or loss, mood swings, and reproductive problems, can be brought on by hormonal imbalances.

A balanced endocrinology requires a healthy lifestyle, which is crucial. This entails consistent physical activity, a healthy diet, and enough sleep. Deep breathing exercises, yoga, and other stress-reduction strategies can support endocrine function.

A healthy endocrine can also be supported by limiting exposure to environmental contaminants such as pesticides, herbicides, and plastics.

It is critical to get a diagnosis and treatment options from a healthcare provider if you think you may have an endocrine imbalance. Depending on the underlying causes of the imbalance, treatment may require dietary adjustments, hormone replacement therapy, or other medical measures. You can improve your health and stave off different endocrine-related conditions by keeping balanced endocrinology.

Balance the endocrine system.

A complex network of glands and organs called the endocrine system creates and secretes hormones, which are chemical messengers that control a variety of bodily processes like growth, metabolism, reproduction, and stress response. The optimal generation and secretion of hormones is the outcome of a balanced endocrine system, which is defined as the proper operation and interaction of the various endocrine system components.

The hormones are created and released in the right amounts and at the right times when the endocrine system is in balance. For preserving good health and preventing diseases, this balance is crucial. Hormone imbalances can be caused by a variety of things, including underlying medical disorders, drugs, lifestyle choices, and heredity. Many symptoms, such as weariness, weight gain or loss, mood swings, and problems with reproduction, can result from these imbalances.

A healthy lifestyle, including frequent exercise, balanced food, and enough sleep are necessary to maintain a normal endocrine system. The endocrine function can also be supported by controlling stress levels and limiting exposure to environmental contaminants. It is crucial to seek medical advice from a qualified practitioner for a diagnosis and treatment options if you think you may have an endocrine imbalance. Depending on the underlying cause of the imbalance, treatment may require dietary adjustments, hormone replacement therapy, or other medical measures.

Endocrine system equilibrium is essential for general health and well-being, to sum up. A person's physical and mental health can be improved, and numerous endocrine-related illnesses can be avoided, by encouraging normal hormone production and secretion.

Chapter 2.

The Endocrine System: What Does It Do.

Endocrine glands produce hormones in the bloodstream. As a result of this, the hormones can now reach cells throughout the body.

The regulation of mood, development, metabolism, and reproduction is aided by endocrine hormones.

The endocrine system regulates how much of each hormone is released.

This may be influenced by the number of hormones already present in the blood as well as other blood components like calcium.

The various things that might impact hormone levels include stress, illnesses, and changes in the fluid and mineral balance of the blood.

Every hormone has a safe and toxic range for the body.

Several of these problems are treatable with medicine.

Which of the following represents a direct interaction between the endocrine and neurological systems?

An illustration of how the endocrine system interacts directly with the nervous system is the hypothalamic-pituitary-adrenal (HPA) axis. The complex feedback loop known as the HPA axis is made up of the hypothalamus, pituitary, and adrenal glands located atop the kidneys.

In reaction to a stressful situation, the hypothalamus sends a signal to the pituitary gland to release adrenocorticotropic hormone (ACTH). After passing through the bloodstream and arriving in the adrenal glands, the stress hormone cortisol is then produced by those structures.

Cortisol assists the body's response to stress by increasing blood sugar, lowering immunity, and speeding up metabolism. Moreover, cortisol can affect the brain, influencing decisions and responses to stress.

The HPA axis serves as an example of how the neurological system and endocrine system work together to react to a stressor. When a stressor is present, the brain sends a signal to the pituitary gland, which subsequently creates a hormone that triggers the adrenal glands to release cortisol. This synchronized response allows the body to react to stress and preserve homeostasis.

What Constitutes the Endocrine System's Components.

Although the body produces hormones throughout, the following glands make up the majority of the endocrine system:

- hypothalamus

- pituitary \sthyroid \sparathyroids

- pineal body and adrenals

- that organ

- the gonads

The pancreas is a component of both the endocrine and digestive systems. This is because it generates and secretes hormones into the bloodstream, as well as enzymes into the digestive system.

The lower central portion of the brain contains the hypothalamus, which is pronounced hi-po-THAL-uh-mus. It links the endocrine and neurological systems. Chemicals produced by nerve cells in the brain regulate the release of hormones made by the pituitary gland. Sensations generated by the brain (such as temperature, light exposure, and feelings) are collected by the hypothalamus and sent to the pituitary. The ability of the pituitary gland to produce and release hormones is impacted by this knowledge.

Pituitary.

In the base of the brain is the pituitary gland, which is about the size of a pea and is pronounced puh-TOO-uh-ter-ee. The pituitary is frequently referred to as the "master gland," despite its diminutive size. Numerous other endocrine glands are controlled by the hormones it produces.

The pituitary gland produces a variety of hormones, including

Growth hormone, which promotes the growth of bone and other body structures and helps the body use nutrients and minerals

The hormone prolactin, which increases milk production in nursing women, is pro-LAK-tin.

Thyrotropin, pronounced "thy-ruh-TRO-pin," stimulates the production of thyroid hormones; corticotropin, pronounced "kor-tih-ko-TRO-pin," stimulates the production of certain hormones by the adrenal gland; and antidiuretic hormone, whose effects on the kidneys help control the body's water balance.

Oxytocin, pronounced "ahk-see-TOE-sin," causes the uterus to contract during labor.

Neurotransmitters known as endorphins, which are also made by the pituitary, function in the nervous system to diminish pain perception. Moreover, the pituitary secretes hormones that tell the reproductive system to create sex hormones. The pituitary gland controls ovulation and the menstrual cycle in females.

Thyroid.

Pronounced THY-Royd, the thyroid is a gland that is situated in the front of the lower neck. Its shape is like a butterfly or a bow tie. Thyroid hormones triiodothyronine and thyroxine are produced by it (pronounced: try-eye-oh-doe-THY-ruh-neen). These hormones control how rapidly food is converted by cells into fuel for energy. The amount of thyroid hormone in the bloodstream affects how quickly various bodily chemical reactions occur.

The growth and development of children's and adolescents' bones, as well as the brain and nervous system, depend on thyroid hormones.

Parathyroids.

Parathyroids are a group of four small glands that are connected to the thyroid and cooperate (pronounced: par-uh-THY-roydz). They release parathyroid hormone, which works with thyroid-produced calcitonin (pronounced kal-suh-TOE-nin) to regulate the amount of calcium in the blood.

Adrenal Glands.

These two triangular adrenal glands, which are pronounced "uh-DREE-null," are located over each kidney. The adrenal glands are divided into two divisions, each of which produces a distinct set of hormones and has a distinct purpose:

1. ***The adrenal cortex is the outer portion.*** It produces hormones known as corticosteroids (pronounced cor-tih-ko-STER-oydz), which aid in regulating the body's salt and water balance, reaction to stress, metabolism, immune system, and sexual growth and function.

2. ***The adrenal medulla is located on the inside (pronounced: muh-DUH-luh).*** It produces

catecholamines, including epinephrine (pronounced: kah-tuh-KO-luh-meenz) (pronounced: eh-puh-NEH-frun). Epinephrine, also referred to as adrenaline, increases blood pressure and heart rate when the body is under stress.

Pineal.

The pineal body, also known as the pineal gland, is located in the center of the brain and is pronounced pih-NEE-ul. It releases melatonin, a hormone that may aid in regulating when you go to sleep at night and wake up in the morning.

Chapter 3.

Reproductive Glands.

The primary source of sex hormones is the gonads. Most people are unaware that both men and women have gonads. The testes, or male gonads, are located in the scrotum in males (pronunciation: TES-teez). They release hormones known as androgens, the most significant of which is testosterone (pronunciation: AN-druh-junz) (pronounced: tess-TOSS-tuh-rone). These hormones signal to the body of a male when it is time for puberty-related changes like height and penis growth, voice deepening, and pubic and facial hair growth. In conjunction with pituitary hormones, testosterone also signals to a man's body when it is time to produce sperm in the testes.

The ovaries, or gonads in female slang, are located in the pelvis. They produce eggs and release progesterone and estrogen, which are feminine hormones (pronounced: pro-JESS-tuh-rone). The onset of puberty in girls is influenced by estrogen. A girl will have a growth spurt throughout puberty, enlargement of the breasts, and the beginning of body fat storage in the hips and thighs. The management of a girl's menstrual cycle also involves the hormones estrogen and progesterone. During pregnancy, these hormones are also important.

Pancreas.

The hormones that regulate the amount of glucose, or sugar, in the blood are produced by the pancreas, which is pronounced PAN-kree-us. These hormones include insulin and glucagon. Insulin aids in maintaining the body's energy reserves. This accumulated energy is used by the body for movement and activity as well as to support healthy organ function.

What is a case when the endocrine system and the circulatory system directly interact?

An example of the endocrine system directly interacting with the circulatory system is when hormones are released by the endocrine system, such as adrenaline and cortisol, and these hormones are then carried by the circulatory system throughout the body to interact with organs and tissues.

Chapter 4.

How Can I Help Keep My Endocrine System Healthy Naturally.

To keep your endocrine system in good shape:

- Get plenty of exercise.

- Eat a nutritious diet.

- Go for regular medical checkups.

- Before using any herbal remedies or supplements, consult your doctor.

- Any family history of endocrine issues, such as diabetes or thyroid issues, should be disclosed to the doctor.

When Should I Call the Doctor?

Inform the physician if you:

- even drinking a lot of water, you still feel thirsty

- have to pee often

- have frequent belly pain or nausea

- are very tired or weak

- have a significant weight gain or loss

- have tremors or sweat a lot

- are constipated

- are not growing or developing as expected.

why is the endocrine system slow?

The slowness of the endocrine system is caused by several factors. The fact that hormones are created and released by many organs and glands throughout the body and that it takes time for them to travel through the bloodstream to reach their intended cells and organs is one of the key causes. Furthermore, because the endocrine system frequently functions in a feedback loop, it may take some time for hormones to accumulate to the right levels and notify the body to begin or halt a process.

The fact that many of the endocrine system's actions are controlled by negative feedback mechanisms is another factor contributing to its sluggishness. In a process known as negative feedback, the body creates a hormone or signal to restore equilibrium when it detects that a certain hormone or process is out of balance. The body may need to create multiple cycles of hormones during this process to have the intended effect.

While being slower than the neurological system, the endocrine system is just as vital. Several of the body's vital processes, such as growth, metabolism, reproduction, and stress response, are controlled by hormones. When the endocrine system is in good shape, it supports homeostasis, promotes overall health, and improves the quality of life.

Freshwater shrimp were populations in two distinct ponds—one mercury-polluted and the other unpolluted—with comparable food webs having their levels of mercury assessed. Which of the following best describes the scientific inquiry that would direct this research?

Get an Answer to this, you can keep it for yourself or Kindly share it with us @ smartblistech4@gmail.com.